A Nurse's Medicine Basket

Tools for Compassionate Self-Care

Tina Bradley Gain, CNM, MSN, RN

Contents

In Honor of Nurses

They are the foundation of genuine compassionate care.

Look closely.

They are all around us.

They are everywhere.

This book is dedicated to nurses, the Angels of Healing.

Forever we are Nurses.

Believe in your dreams.
Believe in today.
Believe that you are loved.
Believe that you can make a difference.
Believe we can build a better world.
Believe what others might not.
Believe that you may be that light for someone else.
Believe that the best is yet to be.
Believe in yourself.
I believe in you.

— Kobi Yamada

A Special Thank You

It is with a grateful heart that I acknowledge the many nurses who courageously came forward to share their experiences and insights while I wrote this book. You know who you are. I will always honor your desire for anonymity, just as I honor you for all you are and all you do. We can't even know how profound a difference your voice and your truth have made in nursing, simply by sharing your experiences in this book.

Thank you for your support, honesty, integrity and willingness to be a part of the movement to reignite the nursing profession. We are and forever will be nurses.

Tina Bradley Gain
July 2018

Author's Note: The Story of the Medicine Basket

In many societies, including the various Native American cultures, healers have connected the past with the present through the powerful healing concept of the medicine basket. This connection is the reason for the title, *A Nurse's Medicine Basket.*

Most Native American healing baskets were traditionally carried by women and described as *burden baskets*, based on the belief: "It takes a strong heart to feel compassion for the burdens of others without taking on those burdens as our own." The sacred tools within the medicine basket were also used for self-care and healing. Medicine baskets provided what was needed at any given time and place for a particular person in need of healing.

For the purpose of this book's message, the medicine basket represents a symbolic vessel

3

woven from many strands to create a safe container for healing and for the numerous diverse tools nurses use in their mission as healers. In their role as the compassionate healers of those in need, nurses provide the safe container for patients and self-care.

Today's nurse is a modern day medicine basket filled with caring, knowledge, skills, empathy, compassion, and integrity. Symbolically, nurses weave intentions and histories into the container of life, day by day, strand by strand. The Native American tradition, belief, and a willingness to provide healing care resonate with modern nursing on many levels, specifically, the importance of self-care.

Foreword

After more than 35 years of nursing, I still remember many of my early patients. In my mind I see their faces, and remember their stories, their struggles, their successes, and sometimes their deaths. I also remember really loving my job. Today? Honestly, not so much.

What has changed? Almost everything—except for the patients. They still suffer from the same diseases. Many get well, many don't. Yet a growing number of patients in this generation have become empowered to ask questions and to challenge what may not make sense to them. A few are even empowered to fire their providers.

What about nurses? How have we changed? Are we becoming empowered to ask questions or challenge authority? And, are we ready to fire our bosses or providers?

As a profession, we've talked about nursing burnout for years and much has been written on the subject. Who among us has actually acted to reverse this trend? Do we observe the emerging crop of new nurses and wonder how long they will last?

In *A Nurse's Medicine Basket*, Tina Bradley Gain explores today's culture of nursing in a fresh, bold manner with the goal of improving the practice of nursing from within our ranks. With candid reflections from nurses around the country, Gain captures the mood of today's nurses in such a way that will lead all nurses to nod in agreement. We nurses know the problem, and this book inspires nurses everywhere to act on what we know and stand up, speak up, and take back our sacred vocation.

Charles "Chuck" Ricks, RN
2018

A born caregiver, Mr. Ricks has experienced a celebrated nursing career encompassing a wide variety of service roles including bedside nursing, nursing management, nurse-educator and nursing director. Mr. Ricks recently served as Clinic Director /Advocate for underserved patients prior to retiring in the beautiful Appalachian Mountains after 35 years of diverse nursing experience.

Introduction: I Am a Nurse

If your experiences would
benefit anybody, give them to
someone.

—Florence Nightingale

My nursing career began in July of 1989. I remember receiving the skinny envelope in the mail that proved I'd passed State Boards. From there my emotions took a roller coaster ride. I was elated, relieved, and scared by the overwhelming reality of the responsibility I committed to. "OMG, this is really happening!" I was also filled with an abundance of gratitude to be in a profession known for its service and expertise in providing compassionate, quality, and safe care.

It's now 2018. I have been nursing for most of 29 years, but they've been interspersed with a few years practicing as a Certified Nurse Midwife. Of course, I've seen and experienced a great deal during that time: celebration, moments of tenderness, providing loving care, and knowing both loss and miracles. I also have not so lovely memories of various things like placing or emptying Foley catheters as my bladder feels ready to burst, my stomach growling from hunger ten hours into my 12-hour shift, nightshift flatulence at the most inopportune moments, and drama involving families, staff and physicians.

Why This Book? Why Now?

Have I seen it all? Of course not. But I have stories, and so do you. What I have seen led to the reason for the book and is based on an ever-growing trend among nurses: an inability or reluctance to care for themselves. My intention is to create an awareness of this dangerous trend and the subsequent effect on healthcare.

For the purposes of this book, self-care is defined as meeting our basic needs, including but not limited to rest, nourishment, and adequate attention to necessary bodily functions, which replenish and promote survival. In addition, meeting our physical needs is intricately associated with overall mental, emotional, and spiritual wellness. Within nursing practice, it's not selfish to holistically care for yourself. It is *imperative.*

When did it become the norm for nurses to put their fundamental needs on the back burner when they committed to becoming caregivers? Eating, going to the bathroom, and taking a 15-30 minute break to clear our heads should be required without question in all areas of nursing. Empowering and supporting nurses to meet their basic needs within the workplace emphasizes the purest form of modeling ways to care for the caregiver. Support for a nurse's wellbeing within the workplace facilitates work flow, efficiency, and optimal teamwork.

I hope readers, both nurses and others, will increase their understanding of what current nursing care entails on a daily basis. I want to facilitate much needed change, including proactively healing our healers, while also repairing the current image of nursing.

The book began in my journal, a safe place to voice my growing frustration and discontent, specifically after a week in nursing where circumstances didn't support and enhance my ability — and desire — to provide quality, safe care. After writing page after page in my journal, it was clear I couldn't remain silent any longer. That's when I made the choice to speak out about what I currently observe, hear, and experience in nursing. I hope my work adds to the voice of nurses, as well as making other nurses aware of the need to transform our current nursing mindset, too often based in apathy. But we can empower ourselves and each other through compassionate self-care.

Throughout my years of practice, I have identified ten elements that contribute to a sad and growing trend in the nursing environment. I share these elements in the coming chapters, and you can trust I based these elements on actual experiences, mostly within the hospital setting where the increasing shortage of nurses has a profound and deep, deep impact on nurses' well-being and the care they provide to their patients.

I'm not alone in my concerns about the current state of nursing. Many other nurses have come forward to share thoughts, wisdom, and inspiration that confirm the current nursing climate is not isolated, rare, or confined to certain areas. No, what you see, what I see, is real and present throughout the nation.

Of all the topics I could cover, I narrowed my focus here to ways to help nurses navigate within the changing landscape of our nursing world, and with an emphasis on how to practice compassionate self-care. The time has come to open a dialog amongst ourselves and use each other as sounding boards to stimulate greater thinking about our field.

A Noble Profession

As Florence Nightingale would tell you, nursing is indeed a noble profession. She believed a nurse embodied compassion, caring, self-sacrifice, and a whole lot of patience. I was taught Nightingale's beliefs from my first day of nursing school. Yes, I believe nursing is about compassionate care, but no, I don't believe nursing includes self-sacrifice. In fact, I've come to believe the notion of self-sacrifice has no role in the nursing profession. For several decades, healthcare organizations have idealized this outdated mindset and it's led to devaluing the hub of its healthcare system—nurses. This is why we experience a disconnect and imbalance between what is expected from nursing professionals and the reality of what nurses actually do.

Ironically, Florence Nightingale had some foresight when she stated, *"Were there none who were discontented with what they have, the world would never reach anything better."*

The truth is, I have been "discontented" for quite some time now. The truth is, I love nursing; the truth is, I hate what nursing has become. Because of these truths, I've made a choice to serve my profession by using my discontent. I will use it to become a catalyst to raise awareness about the need to transform the current mindset amongst nurses from apathy to empowerment.

We can start with the premise that nurses have always served a central role—if not the primary role—in providing healthcare to everyone. They treat the sick and they help people of all ages stay well. Nurses often involuntarily sacrifice their own self-care to meet demands of the delivering care in current healthcare environment. As the saying goes, "When the pitcher is empty, there is nothing left to give." All caregivers can tell you that without replenishing themselves, they're unable to confidently and compassionately care for others. However, even knowing that, self-care for nurses is not valued and now is becoming nearly non-existent.

Why should anyone care about this issue? After all, nurses' inability to care for themselves directly affects the patients and eventually the healthcare organization. That's why this trend must stop. *Now.*

A current buzzword in the caregiving community is "compassion fatigue." It is a by-product of caregivers (especially nurses) being unable to adequately care for themselves as they care for others, which then leads to extreme fatigue, burnout, and debilitating illness. I have often wondered what it will take to prevent burnout among our most precious caregivers, nurses.

I believe healthcare systems have taken advantage of an 87% female dominated occupation, a feminine mindset of caring and nurturing, along with the many of decades in which we've lacked powerful nursing leadership. Years ago, hospital administrators subtly began defining nursing roles to meet their corporate needs without much thought to what nursing professionals need. This goes on even though we can easily argue that nurses provide the bulk of patient care.

Sadly, the vulnerable nurse-employees offered little resistance to these changes. Once again, the profession is filled with women, many of whom are single mothers responsible for providing financial stability for their families. Even those with partners are still providing a substantial portion of the household income. Given these circumstances, it's no wonder nurses see few options, which is why they end up accepting unfavorable conditions and tolerating changes inherently wrong for the nursing profession.

In my mind's eye, I can see administrators shaking their heads as they read this, silently whispering, "No, this is not true." I attribute their ignorance to their lack of understanding of the nursing profession itself. Most administrators have business backgrounds, with the corresponding mindset to make money. For some, it means making lots of money. If a CEO or administrator has never experienced being in the patient care trenches, then I suppose we can understand why he or she might lack empathy. However, this blatant lack of empathy and understanding of caregiving has directly led to the issues we see in providing healthcare today.

I remember a time when the majority of hospital CEOs were physicians, who were more likely to see the bigger picture. They often made decisions focused on employee satisfaction, retention and recruitment. Whether they always acted on their knowledge or not, physician CEOs at least knew that when nurses are happy, their patients also are more likely to be well taken care of and happy.

In my experience, physician-run healthcare organizations value an atmosphere where employees are treated like family. As most of us know, that mindset has fallen by the wayside and in its place we have a corporate mentality based in getting more bang for the buck.

On a daily basis, nurses experience:

- Unrealistic, unsafe nurse-to-patient ratios
- Lack of fair compensation and benefits for working long hours without breaks
- Mandatory call
- Mandatory continuing education that does not apply to the nurse's specialty
- Increased non-nursing duties
- An alarming growing trend in violence towards nurses in the workplace

These are only a few of the influences affecting the current climate of nursing. According to the Bureau of Labor Statistics 2015, nurses make up a vital part of the healthcare industry having the highest employment when compared to other healthcare professionals. Despite nurses being valuable assets, administrators continue to take advantage of nurses' passion, compassion, time, and energy without giving thought to valuing their worth — or their needs.

Recognizing Value

We have all encountered burned out nurses or nurses lacking in passion and compassion choosing nursing as a career because of its ability to provide much needed financial stability based on individual circumstances. However, generally speaking, most nurses observe and respond to the needs of others and are compassionate, empathetic, and altruistic souls with heart. There is an inner knowing of *what* to do and *when* to do. We dance well through the ever changing roles throughout our shift. The way I see it, we're the stars of the show. The inability of nurses to implement self-care during any given shift is just another symptom of a healthcare system in *dire* need of healing.

The time has come to recognize that nurses are not a dime a dozen. Nurses are not just warm bodies to fill vacancies caused by unrealistic expectations and demands from healthcare organizations whose primary goal is making money. The spike in the turnover rate of nurses should serve as an alarm, because the current nursing shortage forecasts the dark cloud that hangs over the future of healthcare. Tick-tock, tick-tock. The clock is ticking, healthcare administrators.

Despite the increasing numbers of nurses graduating from nursing schools, the nursing shortage continues, and healthcare administrators continue to play a fundamental role in nursing shortages. Corporate-driven healthcare is based on a business model, not the healing model, which represents a change in foundation of most, if not all, healthcare organizations.

Much of the current dangerous mindset falls squarely on the shoulders of the administrators and bean counters who have created the difficulties affecting the aging workforce.

Because of the current nursing environment and demands, many baby boomers (me included) are ready to retire from the profession earlier than expected. To make matters worse, nursing schools across the nation are turning qualified applicants away due to a shrinking nursing faculty. Coincidentally, nursing school faculty includes many soon-to-retire baby boomers.

The increasing lack of clinical sites in which students are taught hands-on basics is yet another indicator of a system in trouble. Nursing schools may be graduating more nurses, but the reality is young nurses also are leaving the profession at increasing rates. Sadly, some leaving are new or relatively recent graduates. Still others choose to leave bedside nursing to pursue an advanced nurse practitioner degree.

Just the Facts

According to the American Association of Colleges of Nursing's (AACN) report, "2016-2017 Enrollment and Graduations in Baccalaureate and Graduate Programs in Nursing," U.S. nursing schools turned away 64,067 qualified applicants from baccalaureate and graduate nursing programs in 2016 due to an insufficient number of faculty, clinical sites, classroom space, clinical preceptors, and budget constraints. Most nursing schools responding to the survey pointed to faculty shortages as a reason for not accepting all qualified applicants into baccalaureate programs.

As of this writing, the AACN and National League for Nursing issued a statement opposing cuts to nursing in President Trump's FY 2018 Budget proposal, predicting the approval of this budget will "impede growth in the professional nursing workforce and access to care." In a nutshell, the proposed budget nearly eliminates the funding to programs designed to help educate nurses and nurse educators.

One such program is HRSA's Title VIII, which provided programs that ultimately serve the underserved communities by improving access to quality healthcare through the nursing professionals it helps. Fortunately, this program survived the proposed cuts...until next year's budget is reviewed. If future proposed cuts become a reality, it will be a sad day indeed for nurses and those who desire to pursue nursing as a career. Not only will future proposed cuts contribute to the current and forecasted nursing shortage, it also devalues nursing as a profession worth supporting. By extension the cuts continue the on-going issue of lack of access to quality, safe healthcare for patients.

Overloading Today's Nurses

Nurses have always been documenters. However, the documentation requirements continue to become even more burdensome. This means providing actual patient care is coupled with many hours spent on computer documenting, often continuing long after the shift has ended. This contributes to increased fatigue and stress levels among nurses, which inevitably eventually result in dissatisfaction, apathy, and burn-out.

I have seen countless phenomenal, seasoned nurses leave the profession. I have seen nurses just out of nursing school decide the nursing profession is not for them, at least in part based on juggling the demands of acutely ill patients and the rigors of computer charting. Preparing students for computerized charting is a priority in nursing schools today, but new graduates often find they lack the adequate fundamental skills to actually care for patients. Sadly, it is the bedside nurse preceptor of new graduates who bears the weight of teaching necessary skills such as administering injections, inserting catheters, and starting IVs, in addition to the preceptor's responsibilities. Videos and practice on mannequins just doesn't cut it. Nothing replaces actual patient care.

Indeed, most nurses note the significant decrease in their interaction with patients as they attempt to keep up with mandatory charting. They're frustrated with temperamental computer systems, interactive IV pumps, and medication delivery systems. Everything is scanned. Everything is documented at least twice in different areas of the Electronic Medical Record (EMR).Nurses are the primary users of arguably "more efficient" charting, but the process is finely tuned to meet the needs of other disciplines by providing easy access to information they seek.

As for me, I miss paper charting. A lot. And I'm not alone.

What's most unfortunate is that patients are caught in the crossfire of a broken system—and patients understand it's broken. I believe patients and most healthcare providers understand we need changes in our healing system, now so automated we've lost the human element. Nurses are at the heart of the human element, and we need to get back our ability to relate to patients with the humanity that led us to the profession in the first place.

Healthy Nurses: Mind, Body, and Spirit

Keeping our nurses healthy in mind, body, and spirit is the key to creating a healthy healthcare system. The ten elements I explain in this book are intended to provide insight into issues affecting today's nurses and the world of nursing. Nurses always have been agents of change for others, but the time has come for nurses to create positive change for themselves. The benefits of focusing on the overall health of nurses will apply to the profession, patients, and the healthcare system itself. Compassionate self-care will enable nurses to thrive and ultimately survive the demands of our current healthcare system.

In a business-oriented healthcare system focused on the bottom line (yes, that would be money), it is the nurse's *right* (yes, you read this correctly) to practice compassionate self-care and to empower a change in how nursing is perceived and practiced. Nurses also have the right and obligation to be role models of change agents in healthcare.

The healthcare industry has the responsibility to value and *care* for nurses and honor nurses' commitment to patients, along with valuing their expertise, knowledge/education, time commitment, and contributions. Consistently taking care of nurses will go a long way toward the achieving the financial stability healthcare administrators want.

Keeping in mind nursing is both challenging and rewarding, all nurses have a "why" they became a nurse. It seems everyone knows nurses are the front line, so when will nursing professionals be truly recognized for what they bring to the table? The corollary question is equally critical: When will nursing leaders stand strong and courageously say, "Enough!"

At this point in my life, I'm passionate in my belief that it's time for nurses to find the strength, courage, perseverance, and voice to define nursing as we believe it to be: serving our patients and ourselves from a firm foundation of knowledge and experience. I also believe nurses have the ability to change the current mindset within healthcare. We can transform nursing into a respected profession that knows and protects its worth and defines clear expectations for our roles. We can bring nursing to a whole new level to meet the needs of patients, administrations, and especially nurses. Our strength lies in our numbers, in defining our roles, and speaking and standing strong in our truth, and practicing our healing art.

We are nurses.

> *Our human compassion binds us the one to the other—not in pity or patronizingly, but as human beings who have learnt how to turn our common suffering into hope for the future.*
>
> *—Nelson Mandela*

Part I

Using this Book

Bringing about change requires more than one voice, and certainly more than the reach of this single book. We need a growing group of dedicated healthcare professionals, and even patients our invested participants) to discuss, brainstorm, and take action to identify and implement solutions.

At the end of each chapter, you're invited to consider the questions and share the answers, if you'd like. I recommend you have a notebook or specific file on your computer to record your thoughts.

By doing so, you'll provide a record of your growth in your nursing career as well as sparking more questions or solutions… and maybe some "Aha" moments. Begin now to open a discussion about what it means to be a nurse. For now, start with these:

1. What was the experience that led you to answer the call to become a nurse?

2. What emotions did this experience bring to you?

3. Who inspired you to become a healer and why?

The Golden Rule of Nursing: To Thine Own Self Be True

To be yourself in a world that is constantly trying to make you something else is the greatest accomplishment.

—Ralph Waldo Emerson

Define your practice and know your "why." Nursing practice is defined by one's life experiences, desires, personality, and base of knowledge. These "tools" create an individual standard of care provision and expectations, thus enabling nurses to meet the demands of navigating an ever-changing healthcare system without losing themselves in the process. It is most important to ground your practice, because by doing so you're able to meet your own self-care needs. Only you know what fuels your body, mind, heart, and soul. Self-care is *the* foundation and optimal tool in defining your practice. It bears repeating: *If your nursing practice leaves you depleted, you will have nothing to give to others.*

Most nurses follow their calling to become a nurse based on their passion for caregiving. Nursing is a profession of perpetual learning and continual stimulation, which allow for personal and professional growth. We experience gratitude and grace knowing we have met others' needs at their most vulnerable time.

My *why* for becoming a nurse was and continues to be the desire to be present for others, and promoting, empowering, and nurturing healing from within. I am honored to be invited into an individual's time of vulnerability and grateful to be part of a healing experience, whatever that may be. I have been keenly aware since early childhood that nurturing others is my soul's purpose in life. Being a nurturer is at the core of who I am. The "why" is the foundation for your practice and creates passion and the ability to have realistic boundaries.

It's easy for caregivers to fall into the role of a martyr. Believe me, I know. Been there, done that. For example, it's not nurturing the nurturer to stay long past my shift to meet staffing and patients' needs, knowing I have to return for my scheduled shifts the next two days. During that time, all I did was eat, sleep, and work. That is *not* life balance. Ultimately, I was brought back to reality when I realized I was unable to truly nurture and meet my patients' needs if I failed to take care of myself.

I also found myself joining other nurses in a downward spiral created by personnel shortages. I began to decline offers to add hours and days to my scheduled shifts. As more nurses reached the point of depletion and increasingly declined to stay past their shift, many hospital administrators exerted their power and implemented mandatory call. This is a blatant example of dismissing nurses' needs. In addition, their voices were silenced by threats of being fired for abandoning their patients.

It continues to baffle me how organizations are unable to connect the dots. If they honor and care for the nursing staff they're promoting excellent care of the patients, thus reflecting positively on the organization.

Define your Boundaries

Having strong boundaries allows clarity of roles within the healthcare system. As a nurse you have something extraordinary that only you can give to the profession, or you couldn't have survived the rigors of nursing school in the first place.

To place even more emphasis on boundaries, you can't be everything to everybody. Taking on responsibilities that belong to other disciplines within healthcare creates fatigue, resentment, and eventual burnout and/or stress-induced illness. Your body, mind, and spirit will rebel and eventually you'll leave nursing altogether.

Nursing needs you! Know your *why* and consistently measure your practice by your why. Your success in anything you pursue must come from loving what you do. Nursing may not be easy, but it's sure worth it.

We were among the first nursing teams to arrive in Miami after Hurricane Andrew and going door to door looking for bodies — dead and alive. The location was one of the hardest working conditions I have ever encountered. We were guarded by the 82nd Airborne because the area was so unsafe. Eleven of us volunteered for this mission and it was some of the most satisfying and fulfilling work I ever did. This experience showed me nursing was the right profession for me.

— Anonymous, FL

There are days when I sit in the parking lot looking at the entrance of the hospital and ask myself if I really want to go inside. I almost know what the day will bring just looking at the number of cars in the parking lot and I feel dread.

    I don't think of the day as being too much work as much as knowing in my heart at the end of the day, I haven't been able to meet my patients' needs as I would like. That thought saddens me to tears and I wonder why I ever chose nursing as a career. In my heart, what I'm experiencing is NOT nursing.

— Anonymous, PA

On the days you wonder why you ever pursued a nursing career, knowing your why will help keep you grounded and heart-centered, guiding you to make sound decisions that support you, not tear you down.

Moral of the story: If your current place of employment is not aligning with your why, find one that does. Remember your why for nursing. Stand in your truth, in what you believe, and be the gift to nursing you truly are.

> *Our first teacher is our own heart.*
>
> — *Cheyenne proverb*

The Golden Rule Nursing Style

As a child, I wasn't aware of what I now consider to be my golden rule: *To thine own self be true.* As an adult, I've come to understand the complexities of Shakespeare's words from *Hamlet.* As a nurse, this core belief has allowed me to create a standard for myself, a guideline by which I can measure my actions, my choices and the responses of those in my sphere of influence.

Everyone has a core belief that tolls a clear bell when our actions and beliefs are attuned to each other. "To thine own self be true" means to be authentic, to know who you are, to listen to your inner voice, and be free to choose your own path in life.

I have only been a nurse for three years and am completely overwhelmed with four mother/baby couplets. When assigned five mother/baby couplets, I could sit down and cry knowing I cannot give them the care they deserve and appropriately expect from a nurse. Because of the tremendous amount of charting with each additional couplet, I lose more nursing time and believe I'm not truly present for my patients as I would like to be. I can only do the minimum of nursing care and pray to God throughout my shift that I don't make a mistake that could be detrimental to my patients...especially the babies. I do my best under the circumstances, but always leave after my shift believing I didn't do enough.

—Anonymous, NC

An ICU nurse from Pennsylvania relates:

I had been an ICU nurse for two years and had two patients on ventilators with another who needed most of my attention. Because of the instability of this patient's condition, I was concerned that I was not caring adequately for all of my patients and was far from meeting care standards. I was overwhelmed. There was nobody to ask for help because we all had three to four critical patient assignments. It was one of the saddest days in my early nursing career. I almost left nursing after that. I ended up going to a different hospital. It wasn't much better, but still better than what I had left.

—Christina, PA

I guess everyone wants to believe they make a difference. That's why we became nurses, right?

—Jeni, OR

If we don't stand for something, we will fall for anything.

—Irene Dunn, Actress

Thoughts on Your Truth

Consider these questions and share them if you like. Your beliefs, experiences, and thoughts are important.

1. What is your truth and how does it align with the current nursing climate?

2. What role does fear play in being true to yourself in nursing?

3. What is non-negotiable in your practice as a nurse?

Not Always about the Paycheck

> *Your profession is not what brings home the paycheck. Your profession is what you were put on earth to do with passion and such intensity that it becomes spiritual in calling.*
>
> — *Vincent VanGogh*

Nurses are one of the highest-paid professions of our generation. According to the U.S. Bureau of Labor Statistics' "2016-17 Occupational Outlook Handbook," the median national annual salary for registered nurses is $67,490. Yet working in the hospital day in and day out requires more than a fat paycheck. A compassionate heart and willingness to care for a stranger are what nurses need to survive a very demanding career.

I don't think anyone can do this job without loving it. It's a service position in that all you do is give.

— Anonymous, FL

It's not unreasonable to expect a fair wage and financial security in exchange for the passion for nursing, expertise, hard work, and the time and energy nurses expend. Nurses are worth every dollar, yet money is not the prime motivation for most called to nursing. These nurses give 100% because nursing is a passion and giving service as a healer brings abundant fulfillment and joy. Fortunately, it's rare for a fat paycheck to be the primary why for nurses.

Nurses are Human

We all share a desire to be rewarded for effort and to look for the best opportunity for fair remuneration. But a paycheck can't replace the need for the passion and compassion nursing requires. The paycheck alone is not enough to face the ongoing demands of a nursing career day after day.

If your why is defined only in financial terms, the shock of the stressors involved in the job may lead to a short-lived career. This is especially true for the job that dangled a big ass bonus in front of you; it may prove to have more strings attached than what you bargained for. You'll be miserable, your fellow staff members will be miserable working with you, and most of all, your vulnerable patients will be short-changed and miserable as well.

As Steve Jobs so eloquently stated, "Your work is going to fill a large part of your life and the only way to be truly satisfied is great work. The only way to do great work is to LOVE what you do."

Go back to the Golden Rule: *To thine own self be true.* Enough said.

You are Worthy

Speaking of paychecks, here is the "flip side" of the coin (pun intended).

There's no shame in expecting compensation for doing something you love. Know your worth and don't settle for anything less. I learned this lesson when I relocated from one city to another and was told the reason for my significant cut in hourly pay was due to the lower cost of living. I believed the recruiter instead of trusting my gut instinct after researching and comparing the two cities.

As it turned out, the only significant decrease in my cost of living was the price of gas. Yep. That would be it. For the record, the lower cost of living quote did not include being taxed for almost everything in my new state, compared to living in a state with no sales tax. You can imagine I was surprised, dismayed, and disillusioned, not to mention being a little angry with myself for not trusting my instincts.

The sadder part of this story, my nursing friends, is that most of the nurses within this particular healthcare system believe this lower cost of living spiel, because few had worked outside this specific healthcare system. Amazingly, they believe they are fairly compensated since they experience nominal raises—and I mean nominal—as cost of living adjustments.

One nurse who has worked for over thirty years in the South indignantly commented, "Until you Yankees started working here, we never even got a raise." As a native of

Pennsylvania, was I to take that as a compliment? I chose to do so and to research the compensation practices within one specific healthcare organization. I learned its nurses have settled for lack of appropriate compensation for being called back to work within their mandatory call time, paid only their base hourly salary for most holidays and offered nominal "incentive" pay to work past their shift to help cover staffing.

I also have to wonder about healthcare systems that don't acknowledge additional education degrees and reluctantly compensate nurses for their years of experience or certifications. This makes no sense since nurses further their knowledge base with the intention to provide better care to their patients. The negative mindset among administrators doesn't say much for how a specific healthcare organization perceives the value of the nursing staff. Fortunately, not all healthcare systems operate on this level and do appropriately compensate their nurses fairly.

Know your worth. *You* are worth it.

> *It is not how much you do, but how much love you put in the doing.*
>
> *– Mother Teresa*

Thoughts on Knowing and Embracing Self-Worth

Consider these questions and share your thoughts, beliefs and experiences:

1. What true belief do you hold about your worth in nursing?

2. How has your worth been valued as a nurse?

3. What ways do you think would validate your value as a nurse within your current workplace?

You Don't Know Everything...and You Never Will

Let us never consider ourselves finished nurses...we must be learning all our lives.

—Florence Nightingale

One of my nursing school instructors, Kay Fedorka, was an especially wise and professionally savvy nurse. To this day, I remember her words:

It's never a matter of knowing everything in nursing. That's unrealistic. What you need to know is how and where to find the answers.

I took her wisdom to heart and her words have helped me in more ways than I'd have ever imagined. Knowing your resources and where to find accurate, evidence-based information to shape your practice is a *must*.

The longer I'm in medicine, the more I realize I don't know everything.

–Lisa, FL

There is absolutely no way to know everything. Medical science is always changing as new information is discovered and creating new standards of care and modalities. Because of their diverse expertise and knowledge base, nurses are frequently the first to be called upon to *be* the change as well as implement the changes. The pendulum is always swinging. It's in your best interest to be honest with yourself, patients, and colleagues if you don't know the answers. Then look for the answers from various appropriate resources and share! You and your peers learn and patients respect your honesty about what you didn't know and love you for your commitment to find the answers. It's a win-win.

The larger the island of knowledge, the greater the banks of wonder.

—Anonymous

Your responsibility also includes being aware of inaccurate information that can have a detrimental effect for everyone involved. I'm referring to staff members who believe they have all the answers or pass on outdated information.

It takes a lot of courage to call someone out on their lack of accurate knowledge, and the situation is delicate. However, coming from a place of grace, we can be professional at all times, and honor and respect where they are in their current knowledge base. Granted these individuals might not initially appreciate your insights, but you've planted a seed. Perhaps your contribution will open up opportunities for everyone to learn new information that benefits patients.

If the behavior persists, have the courage to talk with your supervisor. It's a mistake to ignore the behavior of a know-it-all. In my experience, lack of accurate observation and deduction result in more mistakes than lack of knowledge.

Never let formal education get in the way of your learning.

— Mark Twain

I worked with a young nurse about four years into nursing who thought she knew everything. Most of the staff found her to be insufferable. Her behavior had been mostly tolerated until the CAUTI Best Practice implementation began where two nurses were required to be present during a Foley catheter insertion.

I was paired with this young nurse and noticed a break in the sterile field. I asked her if she would like another catheter kit, but since we were in the patient's room I didn't mention the break in sterility prior to the actual insertion. She looked at me as if I had three heads and said no.

I proceeded to stop the procedure by making an excuse to have her step outside the patient's room to explain. To make matters worse, the nurse did not go willingly and argued with me in front of the patient.

She became quite upset claiming, "I know how to insert a Foley"

It was so dramatic and it didn't have to be. I felt lucky that after our manager heard both sides, she understood erring on the side of patient safety and maintaining protocol. It took some time before this young nurse would speak to me. It felt like weeks. In my heart, if the shoe had been on the other foot, I would've looked at it as a teaching moment. A gift to change my practice for the better.

It is interesting to note, and not to judge, this nurse is now a nursing instructor for BSN students.

— Anonymous, OR

If we wonder often, the gift of knowledge will come.

— Arapaho

Thoughts on Skills and Knowledge

Consider these questions and share your thoughts, beliefs and experiences:

1. What do you consider your most valuable and dependable resources?

2. Describe an experience within your practice you wish you had handled differently.

3. How do you handle questions or experiences you feel uncertain about?

Part II

Develop Your Voice—You're Gonna Need It

Nurses are a unique kind. They have this insatiable need to care for others, which is both their biggest strength and fatal flaw.

—Dr. Jean Watson, Nursing Theorist

Nursing is not for the faint of heart—and in more ways than I imagined nearly 30 years ago. Nurses are not only a voice for patients. Nurses also, and this is often overlooked, must be the voice for self. This is where the boundaries come in. And the courage to speak your truth.

Admittedly, it took me years to speak up and stand in my truth. For most, having the ability to embrace vulnerability and speak on behalf of yourself, your peers, and your patients takes courage. It also takes time to feel comfortable doing so, because it's no secret healthcare is a field filled with strong personalities.

In healthcare, we see an environment that calls on us to "prove ourselves" to our peers, physicians, and patients. However, in recent years I found the only one I was proving myself to would be me. As a person who is shy and insecure in large groups, the experience of being talked over became the catalyst to find my voice. It took time. I had to learn to communicate clearly and speak from the heart. I also had to be willing to step out through my own and risk receiving criticism from my peers to find that voice. Standing firm in my truth despite the naysayers, the bullies, and know-it-alls took courage, but I found my voice and in the process became firm and less meek.

Can you spell freedom? My career took a whole different turn for the better, specifically in relation to my relationships with peers and physicians, but especially the patients.

More importantly, personal and professional

growth resulting from having (and using) our voices can't be minimized or ignored. Speak up! You may have something to say that could change your unit, your patient's care, and your relationships for the better. What you have to say could be a game-changer for the nursing profession and standards of nursing care. Whether or not anyone agrees with what you have to offer, the point is, you are making a statement of who you are and what you believe.

I believe that all new nurses should have a seasoned nurse as their mentor to model how and when to use their voice, let alone find it. We have all had nasty doctors to deal with. Role modeling from older nurses allows younger nurses to gain the ability to know how and when to pick their battles.

— Anonymous, FL

To be beautiful means to be yourself. You don't need to be accepted by others. You need to accept yourself.

– Thich Nhat Hanh

Here is a true story. I am sad to say that I witnessed this event.

A nurse in a busy labor and delivery unit was called on the carpet, in front of her patient and family no less, by a physician because she had not made certain that the physician's desired shoe covers and mask were available. As the physician ranted on and on, the nurse stood in silence.

The physician decided to go back to the clinic because the patient's pushing efforts were not showing the desired progress the physician expected. The nurse caught the baby fifteen minutes later because the physician didn't make it back to the room in time after being paged to return.

The beauty of this story is the nurse listened to the physician's verbal abuse until it was clear the unacceptable dressing-down was complete. Without hesitation, she made it a point to look directly in the physician's eyes, and calmly said, "I did the best I could do under the circumstances."

Notice she did not apologize, nor did she affirm she was the blame for the physician's lack of judgment, timing, and frustration. She did her job and then some. She maintained her professional composure, unlike that of her colleague. The nurse chose to take the high ground, accepting the physician's frustration was misplaced because of a poor decision he made. The nurse was an easy, if inappropriate, target for the physician's lack of judgment.

This story also has another side — the patient's and family's take on how this situation went down. The patient and her family were visibly upset and spoke out about their disbelief that the physician treated the nurse so poorly. The nurse had established a trusting connection with the family, having met their needs hours prior to the birth of the patient's first baby. The family thought she did her job exceptionally well and were grateful for her expertise and care. Grateful and outraged, the family was compelled to write to the administration and describe what they witnessed.

Talk about reverse advocacy! The patient and family knew who the true professional was in this situation. And, they let it be known to the appropriate entity.

The moral of this story: Speak your truth with professionalism, dignity, compassion and respect for self and conviction.

We are each gifted in a unique and important way. It is our privilege and our adventure to discover our own special light.

– Mary Dunbar, British Artist, Illustrator and Teacher notable for recording contributions of women during WWII

Thoughts on Having a Voice and Being Heard

Consider these questions and share your thoughts, beliefs and experiences:

1. How do you communicate your truth in seemingly hostile situations?

2. In what ways do you stand in your truth despite those who believe otherwise?

3. What is your belief about the best way to be heard in any given situation?

God gives us each a song.

— Ute

Build Up Your Team: Be the Type of Nurse You Want to Work With

A good word is an easy
obligation; but not to speak ill
requires only our silence;
which costs us nothing.

— John Tillotson

It is so very easy to get caught up in the gossip and judgment that circulates within the nursing station. There are three possible actions to consider when choosing to be proactive and build up our team.

1. Walk away and not say a word.

2. Fuel the frenzy of the witch hunt by adding your own thoughts to tearing your co-

worker down.

3. Find compassion for the individual being gossiped about and give her/him a voice in their absence.

Wouldn't it feel much better to be in an environment that built up coworkers versus tearing them down? Wouldn't it feel good to know that someone had your back if you happen to be the target of the gossip mill? I have experienced both sides of the fence. I am no angel and not proud of being one of the participants in gossiping about another. As the old saying goes, "What goes around comes around." Yep, I've also felt the sting of being gossiped about. Ow! Both experiences have helped me learn to make every effort to avoid the abyss of choice number two for the sake of all involved.

We have enough stress in our profession without having others chip away at *perceived* imperfections of another person within our team. Gossip creates distrust and alienation. As children we knew it hurt, and as adults it still hurts, but we minimize the damage. Besides, most gossip is based in assumption and things that aren't true, as well as insecurity.

What does it say about a profession that

purports to place compassionate care at the top of their philosophy when they are unable to have compassion and kindness towards one another?

Granted there are times when a team member needs to be called out on bad behavior that negatively affects the department and reflects badly on it. For example, we need to stand up to a bully, and we have ways to do it with kindness, respect, and compassion. We can actively choose to hold true to a firm statement of intolerance of bullying in the workplace. I've seen this kind of behavior modeling used to stop abhorrent bullying behavior. Without participating allies, bullies all but lose their power.

To be honest, I don't believe there is a nurse out there who has not experienced some form of bullying during their career, and I include myself. According to a study by RNnetwork (a travel nursing company), more than half of nurses are currently considering leaving the profession. This study reports the following alarming statistics based on nursing input:

- 45% of nurses have been verbally harassed or bullied by other nurses
- 41% of nurses have been verbally

harassed or bullied by managers or administrators

• 38% of nurses have been verbally harassed or bullied by physicians.

C'mon folks, we're professionals. We must walk the talk and support one another despite any animosity during our shifts as we work towards providing exceptional care. Be remarkable at providing exceptional care to your co-workers. As William Thackeray sweetly recommended: *Never lose a chance of saying a kind word.*

A young nurse, who has been in the nursing profession just shy of two years relates:

I feel as if there is a bulls-eye on my back. I can't do anything right! I'm more angry than hurt about this." I would've welcomed the feedback to improve. It's too hard to come to work and wonder who I can trust. Who has my back?

All I want to do is give my patient's good care. I have no choice but to leave. I cannot grow in an environment like this.

Invent your world. Surround yourself with people, color, sounds, and work that nourish you.

—Susan Ariel Rainbow Kennedy (SARK)

Of course, there are three sides to any story—yours, mine, and the truth. However, within the young nurse's words we see elements of truth interspersed with her vulnerability and the need to be nurtured early in her career. This example is yet another facet of nursing we could manage with compassion, guidance, understanding, and reasonable expectations for her skill level.

According to HealthStream research, 31% of new nurses leave after the second year. HealthStream is a corporation dedicated to improving patient outcomes through the development of healthcare organizations' employees. The company is contracted by healthcare organizations throughout the United States for workforce development, training &

learning management, talent management, credentialing, privileging, provider enrollment, performance assessment, and managing simulation-based education programs. They also focus on research-based solutions to healthcare organizations' ability to meet standards of care.

This young nurse left her unit. She chose to stay with her profession and to consider this part of learning. She took an honest look at the situation and realized that change was needed....first with her role in this situation. She owned her truth and was ready to "make it good." She was a girl after my own heart when she said with great resolve:

I am going to make this situation something that no nurse will ever experience on my watch. I'm pissed off and I'm going to make a difference modeling kind behavior towards my fellow nurses. Bullying will never be tolerated when I'm around."

— Anonymous (State omitted per request)

The fire in her words confirmed her desire to change this experience into something positive. No self-pity for this young nurse. She was on target with the desire to create an environment that nurtures and supports *all* nursing staff.

I commend her for taking the courage and strength to do what she felt in her heart was the right action to take. She chose to learn and grow from her experience. Watch out for this one. You will be hearing about her advocacy for her beloved nursing comrades. As she lovingly cares for her patients, she also lovingly cares for her fellow nurses as well.

Speaking of patients, they watch and listen. Most patients notice — and note — the interactions between nursing staff members. They recognize even subtle disapproval or animosity between staff members. Bedside reports as well as the conversations at the nurses' station provide a glaring spotlight for patients to observe how the staff interacts with one another.

Be aware of the consequences of gossiping about nursing co-workers at the nurses' station and treat your colleagues as you would like to be treated at the bedside. If you choose to talk smack about your co-workers, the patient's bedside is certainly not the place to undermine your fellow nurse's credibility or skills.

These situations usually occur with a small number of nurses I call *"Repeat Offender Nurses."* This subset of nurses develops a pattern of behavior that capitalizes on the vulnerability of new hires and less experienced nurses. Repeat Offender Nurses strive to control other nurses and through undermining and sabotage they maintain their self-perception of superiority and bolster their claim to be experts among the staff. Unfortunately, I have observed this phenomenon in every nursing unit I've known.

When patients witness such interactions, they see unprofessional, insecure, mean-spirited behavior and the kind of nurse no patient would want caring for them or their family. This behavior also results in patients becoming confused and insecure about the care they are receiving. I have witnessed the aftermath of this type of communication and it isn't pretty.

Here's a newsflash for Repeat Offender Nurses (and if you are honest, you know who you are): You hold a false belief. A new nurse is not made stronger if they survive your test of fitting in. The definition for this abhorrent behavior is bullying and it needs to stop. You are not only hurting yourself. You are hurting your fellow nurses. You are hurting the nursing profession. *Stop*.

Choose to support rather than judge. Condemning the nurses you work with cannot build a strong, cohesive bridge between existing team members and new nurses. It is caring and respectful behavior within the healthcare team that delivers a definitive, powerful statement of, "I care and I've got your back."

Furthermore, cohesiveness has a ripple effect reaching the patient and family and reflects a healthcare team that knows the definition of compassionate care. This leaves no doubt in a patient's mind about the ability of staff to provide care in a manner that reflects the way they care for each other.

It's all about the team you work with. Assigned teams work together to contribute their best talents in any given situation. Working in assigned teams meant that when you were all there, the team could make the best of any bad situation.

It doesn't matter if you're weak or strong in any given area. Everyone in the team makes a difference and learns to work well together.

—Anonymous, FL

Do not judge your neighbor until you walk two moons in his moccasins.

— Cheyenne Proverb

Thoughts on Building a Team and Bullying

Consider these questions and share your thoughts, beliefs and experiences.

1. What choices do you make to build up your team?

2. What action(s) do you choose when confronted with an opportunity to hear (or share) a bit of juicy gossip?

3. How do you handle bullying as a witness or recipient?

Ask For Help

Coming together is a beginning; keeping together is progress; working together is success.

—Henry Ford

You will find your strength in teamwork. A nursing team is only as strong as the weakest link; in practical terms this means experienced nurses must support the weaker nurses, who are most likely the new graduates. After all, when nurses retire, who will take up the baton to continue the race if we don't have new grads ready to learn the art of nursing?

This also means new grads must ask questions. When you ask for help and support, experienced nurses respect your willingness to show your vulnerability. This willingness to learn is part of what assures your success in nursing.

As nurses get older they mature and realize they don't have to do it all. Younger nurses feel like that they have to do it all and are afraid to ask for help because they believe they will be judged incompetent by their peers. They also feel the need to prove themselves and will do anything they are asked.

— Anonymous, FL

Most nurses feel 'incapable' if they ask for help. This is an ego thing. They need to get over it and ask. Otherwise, the patients lose. Always.

— Anonymous, FL

Once I learned I wasn't alone, that was when I knew I was comfortable in the ICU unit.

— Anonymous, FL

To seasoned nurses, *be* the leaders in modeling good behavior through nurturing and supporting *all* your teammates, and in doing so, your unit will be as strong and resilient as Fort Knox.

Since not one nurse knows it all, we must come together as a team. We each bring our individual gifts to the table, share what we know, and ask for help to fill in the gaps. There is no shame in asking for help.

And, if you sense shaming or judgment from another nurse, use the opportunity to tell the nurse how you feel. She just might be having a rotten day and didn't realize how she was coming across. Use this experience to shift your thought processes, and those of your coworker, to benefit your unit. Everyone in your team needs to agree it's okay to expect to receive help.

A strong team leader is important. If you're working with bitchy nurses, you're not going to ask them for help because you feel vulnerable and judged. An alert team leader will pick up on this and step in to help without being asked. Strong team leaders have the ability to teach others how to positively facilitate an environment that is less democratic.

—Anonymous, FL

Be the one to make a difference, and you'll leave a memorable impression on that particular nurse and others. Demonstrate how you expect to be treated within your department. It's important to know that you will be treated by others the same way you treat yourself. Be kind, respectful, compassionate and loving towards yourself and others will follow your example.

Nursing has changed dramatically as a profession, but it survives and prospers today with one strong commonality that spans the ages. Nurses, by any definition, are a group of individuals connected by the common goal of caring. There is no room for lone wolves in nursing. We need each other in more ways than can be counted, and the success of the nursing professional relies on the sum of all the elements and individuals that form the whole.

Our profession will truly be successful when individuals unite around a common cause based in kindness and compassion for self and each other. We each have the opportunity to heal the heart, mind, soul, and body of our patients, their families, and ourselves.

I recall one patient whose husband was noticeably moved by the nursing staff's response when his wife experienced complications related to her hospital stay. He shared this with me:

Our primary nurse was phenomenal and made us feel safe and well cared for despite what was going on. My wife and I were so scared. Almost immediately after our nurse called for help, five other nurses came into the room. It was amazing to watch how smoothly and professionally each nurse in our room contributed to resolving the situation. They communicated calmly, quietly, clearly and formulated a plan right on the spot! We are forever grateful because that group of nurses knew what to do as they worked together to stabilize my wife even before the doctor arrived. I am truly amazed.

Another example came when a newly hired young nurse was finishing her orientation. She was nervous and clearly not certain if she was ready to be on her own. She related to me later:

I had this experience on my last day of orientation that gave me the awareness that although I don't know everything, I do know that my current co-workers have my back. All I did was call out for help and three nurses came to assist me. They made me feel that I mattered. They nurtured me and confirmed that I made the right decision taking this nursing position. I feel so lucky.

— Anonymous, NC

On the flip side of the wonderful experience is a true story of another recent new nursing graduate who felt overwhelmed to tears. In fact, she cried as she shared her story with me, still uncertain about her career choice:

I'd only been on the unit a few weeks and it felt like I couldn't do anything right in my preceptor's eyes. I would cringe when I had to ask her for help and then could hear her audible sigh as she rolled her eyes. I don't think I'm cut out for this. Nursing isn't what I thought it would be.

— Anonymous, NC

To Nursing Preceptors

Please remember your humble beginnings. We all began in nursing inexperienced and at best partially trained. Granted, some come to the floor better trained than others. Ours is a profession that never finishes training and our experience is gained on the job with live patients. This will not change. The challenges around providing nursing care always involve the unique needs of each patient. New nurses rely on learning from you.

Nurture, respect, and be grateful to the new grads with the smarts and courage to recognize they are out of their comfort zone and asking for your expertise. They seek mentorship. They seek invaluable advice and help that can come only from sharing your many years of experience. That, my nursing friends, is a true teaching moment for both you *and* your orientee.

At times, the preceptor and orientee relationship is not a good fit, usually because of personality differences. Since this kind of relationship results in unnecessary stress, it's up to the experienced nurse to know when to call it quits and find another preceptor better suited for the orientee's personality.

It is not your failure—it isn't really about you at all. Committing to be a preceptor comes with the responsibility of knowing what's in your orientees' best interests, even if it means finding a better fit for them. You're in a position to make a difference at the start of a new grad's career...for better or worse.

They may forget your name,
they may forget what you did,
but they will never forget how
you made them feel.

– Maya Angelou

I have seen that in any great
undertaking, it is not enough
for a man to depend simply on
himself.

—Lone Man, Teton Sioux

Thoughts on Mentorship and Professionalism

1. What experiences as a new grad contributed to your nursing practice?

2. What preceptor qualities support you as a nurse?

3. How did you resolve a situation where you experienced a preceptor not meeting your expectations?

Who is the Patient?

*Computers are magnificent
tools for the realization of our
dreams, but no machine can
replace the human spark of
spirit, compassion, love, and
understanding.*

—Louis V. Gerstner, Jr.

Here's a newsflash: The Electronic Medical
Record (EMR) monitor is not, I repeat not, your
patient. It's is no secret I take issue with the EMR
system. I believe the advent of electronic medical
records has dehumanized nursing to a point it
seems nurses are caring for the computer more
than the actual human patient. Speaking for

myself, I feel the joy of nursing sucked right out of me by the end of a twelve hour shift documenting on that damn digital chart.

It makes my head spin trying to keep up with my charting and continue my two decade plus practice of actually looking at and into my patient, observing demeanor, actively listening to the patient's concerns, and touching the patient. If I remember correctly, the nurse's relationship is with the patient. How can one look *into* (not just at) patients when the computerized charting limits our ability to connect with a patient?

One former colleague who is now a nurse manager relates:

My assistant nurse manager and I were talking the other day. We are seeing nurses within our staff who are uncomfortable engaging in more than a superficial conversation with patients. Whatever happened to the belief in honoring 'privileged intimacy'? When did nursing become a profession of being technically proficient? There is a human being in that bed. Being a nurse means having the ability to provide care in the face of vulnerability for our patients' and their families' experiences, as well as having gratitude for being asked into their intimate and private world. We have a responsibility to be present for our vulnerable patients and to provide holistic care.

—Melissa, OR

On another related note, I can't begin to count how many times I've seen nurses charting at the nurses' station versus in their patient's room. Undoubtedly, you'll engage with your patients and their families if you're are in the room. You'll also get a quick intuitive hit on the dynamics within the room as well as your patient's condition.

Time spent at the nursing station computer can't tell you if your patient is seizing, bleeding out, or crying inconsolably from pain or worse. I understand that sometimes it's necessary to catch up on charting (there is a lot of it) without distraction. I get that. What I can't condone is 80% of the twelve hour shift spent on documentation at the nurses' station.

Nursing certainly isn't like it was back when I first started. Back then, nurses actually cared about the personal touch! I get so tired of walking into a unit and seeing everyone sitting at a computer. Who the heck is in the room with the patient? When was the last time anyone put a hand on a laboring belly? I don't know how I got through all those years of taking care of laboring women without monitors or Dopplers.

— Anonymous (State omitted by request)

Here's a story about a patient to illustrate the importance of being with and seeing our patients. A few years ago, the conditions of both my laboring patient and her baby looked absolutely stellar on the central monitoring system at the nurses' desk and on the actual continual printed external fetal monitoring system in her room. I was in this patient's room most of the twelve hour shift. However, when assessing her physically midway into my shift, I discovered an amount of vaginal bleeding inconsistent with "normal" show, which indicates cervical dilation during labor.

I made the physician aware of the situation and he did a bedside assessment and requested close monitoring. Well, the vaginal bleeding continued to occur, intermittently increasing in amount and clots while mom and baby's vital signs and monitoring appeared perfectly normal to the outside nursing station central monitoring world.

Each subsequent incident was reported to the doctor, who returned to the bedside. Eventually, baby began to exhibit signs that indicated distress and a decision for a non-emergent cesarean section was made at the end of my shift. Fortunately, this was an outcome resulting in a healthy mom and baby.

So, what if I hadn't done charting at the bedside and the abnormal bleeding went unnoticed for hours? Scary thought. It brings home the message that the computer is *not* your patient.

Be ever present for your patient. To live up to this motto translates into predominantly bedside patient care during your shifts. There is no substitute.

It's so corporate now. Crappy staffing ratios and more time is spent charting than actually hands on your patient.

– Oregon RN

Alas, technology, aka Electronic Medical Records, is here to stay, along with other technological devices aimed at making our jobs as nurses "easier." Embracing all the technology within my current nursing practice is difficult, if not overwhelming. That's why I'm grateful for the tech savvy nurses I work with who help me understand the intricacies of a system that seems awkward and counterproductive. However, when I listen to my younger nursing coworkers speak of their own frustration with computerized charting, I'm convinced it's not my age or lack of technological skill that leads to frustration. The system itself creates unnecessary stressors within the workplace.

Charting is a waste of time. If a lawsuit results, it's almost impossible to find and decipher what really happened. Charting is not user friendly to obtain the information you need quickly. The issue is that the information is documented as fragments due to all the different places we are required to put it in EMR. You never get the big picture. Documentation is easily overlooked, and it is easy to make a mistake checking boxes. I could not defend myself in a court of law if it came to that. Give me paper where I can adequately document exactly what happened in one place.

— Anonymous, FL

Here's a thought. Although there is a place for technology within healthcare, there is also a place for compromise. This is where nurses need to put their foot down and say no to needless documentation within the EMR to make other disciplines work easier. If the same information is required to be documented in three different places, would not auto-populating the same information provide increased efficiency in the EMR documentation, and also result in less frustration for the nursing staff as they meet mandatory guidelines? If the data are not medically significant, why is it necessary for each department to obtain the same information in various other required areas within the chart? Seems to me the benefits of auto populating redundant information would be a no-brainer in this tech-savvy world.

Perhaps having more IT trained nurses develop the software would allow us to meet the specific charting needs of each individual unit more effectively, while providing an easier charting experience for nursing.

Here's another thought. Create a specific position to address all the non-nursing information mandated by government agencies. I, for one, would like to understand how busy clinical and bedside nurses became the vehicles for providing demographics, among other resources, to non-nursing agencies.

The solution? To begin with, hire a nurse to specifically gather the information healthcare organizations need to meet mandated policies that lead to increased reimbursement. Yes, it would cost money, but in the long run, decreasing their already burdensome load of computer charting would result in greater retention of nursing staff.

So, pulling these thoughts together, I believe the EMR should be making our job and documentation easier, but that's not what has happened. In reality, the EMR takes more time away from patients, has increased nurses' frustration and stress levels, and has decreased, if not depleted, the energy levels of the nursing staff. This, in turn, leads to dissatisfaction, burnout, and turnover.

In my opinion, the mandated hourly rounding documentation is a prime example of fear-based charting to provide evidence of maintained patient safety in an effort to avoid readmissions. I recognize that readmission raises costs for healthcare organizations and also opens them to legal issues. What I don't understand is why the solution to this potential problem falls on the nurses who are already overloaded with increased patient acuity and borderline, if not completely unsafe nurse to patient ratios.

Mandated, unrealistic charting leads to, dare I say, temptation to just click yes because you have to, not because you were actually in the room. How can you honestly say you were in four rooms or more rooms at the same time? I, for one, believe it is unethical and I wouldn't have a leg to stand on in a court of law if I documented I was in room A when I was tied up in room B when room A had a mishap. It is yet another example of charting action put on nurses that really is meant to ease the workload of others within the healthcare system at the expense of quality nursing care.

I wonder if anyone else has given any thought to this issue. Management is well aware of and can actually access how much time is spent in a patient's room through nursing locators and computer log-ins and log-offs.

There are way too many have-to-dos that need not be on our already too full to-do list. Is that really the "why" of what called us to nursing? It certainly isn't my why and never will be.

You treat a disease: You win, you lose. You treat a person, I guarantee you win—no matter the outcome.

—Patch Adams

The frog does not drink up the pond in which it lives.

—Native American Proverb

Thoughts on Technology and Patient Care

1. What are your thoughts on mandated charting?

2. How has electronic charting had an impact on your practice or ability to provide nursing care?

3. What solution(s) would you recommend for computerized charting relative to nursing?

Compassionate Self-Care

*Rest and self-care are so
important. When you take
time to replenish your spirit, it
allows you to serve others
from the overflow. You cannot
serve from an empty vessel.*

—Eleanor Brownn

Compassionate self-care is of the utmost importance. You've certainly heard this many times over the past decade and even longer. Perhaps many resist accepting this innate wisdom because it's become a cliché. Unfortunately, it's also one of the most ignored concepts in our nursing environment.

The current nursing climate doesn't consistently provide ways to practice compassionate self-care. Many of us cling to our innate desire and ability to love and care for others while putting our own needs secondary. This habit of thought most likely results from social conditioning, primarily directed to women.

Let's be clear: *Self-care is not selfish.*

Caring for yourself is an act of survival. As a nurse, it's ever so important to know how to care for yourself. We don't typically have time for self-care during our shifts. We face a fast-paced environment, increased patient acuity coupled with unrealistic nurse to patient ratios. We care for patients' and families' needs and make exhausting efforts to maintain an efficient, steady workflow. At times, we go without bathroom breaks and are unable to get away from the unit for legally mandated (in most states) 30-minute lunch breaks, while becoming physically, emotionally, mentally, and spiritually drained.

Taking care of yourself doesn't mean me first, it means me too.

— *L.R. Knost*

Placing your needs behind your patients' and everybody's needs increases the risk of liability. After all, you're far more likely to become apathetic or make a mistake when your basic needs aren't met.

Instead of accepting things as they are, pair up or find a few buddies and work together to take lunch breaks away from the nurses' station. By the way, eating at the computer doesn't constitute a break. Remember, you're not getting paid for that lunch break. So take it!

If you are unable to take your break, be certain to add "no lunch" when clocking out. It's only a matter of time before word gets out nurses are not getting any real breaks during their shifts and the administration has to explain why. Bottom line: It's not entitlement; it's your *right* to have a lunch break. If you notice team members are running breathless all over the unit, help them to get a break. Others will appreciate your thoughtfulness, and the nurses will learn from it and pay it forward.

Self-care is non-existent with nurses because most are giving it all away and end up having nothing left for themselves. I think a lot of this is because most nurses are co-dependent.

— Anonymous, FL

The ability to say no seems to be quite difficult for most nurses. Work/life balance is the optimal quality of living. Nurses work hard and need to take time to play whether it is during the shift or on your own time. However, if you plan on having a late night with the girls or whoever, please plan it on a night when you don't have to work the next day. Fatigue throughout the day coupled with few or no breaks during the shift and a heavy patient load is not self-care. Learn to say no to situations that impact your self-care.

That said, have the courage to say no to unrealistic assignments, or situations such as staying after work for non-mandatory meetings. Consistently working over-time for little compensation isn't worth your time and energy, take away from valuable sleep time and personal or family time. If you're asked to do something and your first thought is no then say so!

Work/Life balance is important. Learning to say no is important. Home life is important. As nurses, we don't treat ourselves well. Learn self-care when you are young.

— Anonymous, FL

It's not selfish to love yourself, take care of yourself, and to make your happiness a priority. It's necessary.

—Mandy Hale

The American Nurses Association (ANA) recently released the 2017 Code of Ethics for Nurses with Interpretive Statements. These statements are designed to guide nurses in their daily practice in all settings. Interestingly, this book also provides guidance for individual care of the nurse.

Interpretive Statement 5.2 states that, *"Nurses should model the same health maintenance and health promotion measures that they teach and research, obtain healthcare when needed and avoid taking unnecessary risks to health or safety in the course of their professional and personal activities."*

Okay. That sounds well and good—downright logical.

The statement further relates, *"...nurses should commit to eating a healthy diet, exercising and getting sufficient rest in order to balance a satisfying work environment with individual health and well-being."*

I agree with both statements in theory.

When working their shifts, nurses seldom, if ever, have a chance to sit down away from the unit and have a 30-minute lunch let alone consistent bathroom breaks. They're busy providing care with overwhelming nurse to patient ratios, as well as maintaining their documentation with increasingly patient acuity.

It would make more sense for the ANA —a nursing governing body—to advocate, promote, and secure consistent self-care in the workplace, in addition to defining the ideal work environment and practices.

Acknowledge, accept, and honor that you deserve your own deepest compassion and love.

—Nanette Mathews

Compassion is the foundation for the nursing profession. Nurses are held in high esteem for their intelligence, empathy, and hands-on healing abilities. But, it is their *compassion* for others that allows them to hear their call to nursing. As nurses, we have abundant compassion for others. The question is how much compassion do you have for yourself?

Nursing is demanding, even outside of the patient care workload. Nurses handle on-going expectations from licensing boards, patients and families, administrators, educators, peers, and our very own inner critic/desire to validate our worth within an imperfect environment.

Administrators still think they can make good decisions about the things that go on in the hospital without listening to the people who actually do the job. For administration, it's all about the image instead of what is really happening. They really don't give a shit about the patient. It's all about image, projection, and those administrators believe in image rather than the reality.

— Anonymous, FL

Think about how many roles you play in a 12-hour shift. The expectations/perceptions from other disciplines relative to your role as a nurse are…dare I say…unrealistic.

Nurses role-play like no other healthcare professional and are adept at changing hats at any given moment at the dictate of circumstances. Having compassion for yourself is imperative for understanding that no matter how many hats you wore and took off during the day, *you are enough.*

We take very little care of ourselves being our own worst critics. There is very little room for error in nursing. Something most people never have to live with. There have been so many times I found myself waking up in the middle of the night out of a sound sleep wondering if I had set the right IV dopamine drip rate or something else. I didn't realize how

stressed out I was all of the time until I left nursing.
— Anonymous, FL

> **When you have learned**
> **compassion for yourself,**
> **compassion for others is**
> **automatic.**
>
> **—Henepola Gunaratana**

TRUTH: You are not perfect.

No one is perfect. Relationships are not perfect. This is not a perfect world. The current healthcare world we work in is far from perfect. We experience this truth every day even if we don't acknowledge it.

What if imperfection was accepted and viewed as perfection? Let's shift our perception and understanding of what the word imperfection means. The word imperfection breaks down into two words: "I'm Perfection." Yes. You are perfect just the way you are...warts and all.

During our lifetime, we experience multiple imperfections, which society perceives as failures. It is ironic that once we get past of the fear of imperfection, these so called failures allow for professional and personal growth and becoming who we really are,

Any person, nurse or not, who believes perfection is the ultimate goal, may experience an inability to move forward in anything desired in life. Chronically seeking perfection — especially in nursing — creates exhaustion, burn-out, and depression affecting all areas of life.

Don't confuse excellence with perfection. We rarely. if ever. achieve perfection, but we can achieve excellence.

You are enough are three words that can change your life.

> **Lighten up on yourself. No one**
> **is perfect. Gently accept your**
> **humanness.**
>
> **— Deborah Day**

To quote author and speaker, Steve Maraboli and other sages going back to Aristotle, "The most powerful relationship you will ever have is the relationship with yourself." If you are showing up and doing your very best with every situation that presents itself, you are enough. Compassion for self comes when we, as nurses, acknowledge our weaknesses as well as our strengths. Have the courage to unconditionally love yourself as you are.

Having an honest relationship with self gives you the insight and ability to care for others with the same kindness, compassion, and empathy with which you treat self. We are all responsible for our actions. It is up to you how to grow on a professional and personal level. Show up. Do your best. The way you care for your patients is a direct reflection of your relationship with yourself.

A patient recovering from a stroke commented about her experience relative to the nursing care she received:

As I watched the nurses, day in and day out, during my rehabilitation, I saw they were definitely understaffed and working hard to meet their patients' needs. I remember thinking that the nurses are the ones who really know what's going on. One nurse treated me like family. As if I were her child, she'd tuck me into bed each night and made sure all my needs were met and I was comfortable. It made all the difference in my recovery to know a stranger loved me as if I was her own child when I was most vulnerable.

— Jane, NJ

You must love yourself before you love another. By accepting yourself and fully being what you are, your simple presence can make others happy.

— Unknown

You already possess everything necessary to become great.

— Crow

Thoughts on Compassionate Self-Care

1. What "imperfections" have actually turned out to be your greatest strengths?

2. In what ways do you nurture self in your personal and professional life?

3. How do you role model compassionate self-care in your work environment?

Compassion for Management

If you want others to be happy, practice compassion. If you want to be happy, practice compassion.

— *Dalai Lama*

Given that all nurse managers are not created equal, there are two truths when it comes to nurse managers and the staff they direct.

Truth Number One

We have all had nurse managers that made our heads spin like Linda Blair's in "The Exorcist," sans the pea soup projectile vomiting. This management "style" emphasizes behavior consistent with controlling, unpredictability, unclear expectations, biased discipline and disrespectful behavior laced with public humiliation to shame and/or guilt the object of their displeasure into conforming. The nurse tied to the whipping post feels no flexibility, voice, or advocacy and learns quickly not to expect it. There is a disconnect with no effort to heal the breakdown in the relationship. Or perhaps you have experienced a palpable lack of presence for staff when you need a leader.

I am primarily speaking of nursing managers/leaders who are not physically or emotionally available for the nursing staff. This behavior becomes obvious when the nurse to patient ratio has become blatantly unsafe and the manager chooses to remain in the office or go to meetings instead of providing assistance with patient care. Needless to say, such behavior from management, condoned by administration, leaves a nursing unit depleted, devalued and apathetic.

The unit is drowning in a fear-based atmosphere of walking on eggshells and a belief of "not being or doing enough" after working a shift. All too soon, each nurse will begin to believe the inner mean nurse critic's taunting, and will accept the idea of not being enough. This mind-set results in nurses who second-guess and question their ability and knowledge, along with their call to the profession of nursing.

Forget about paddles for the canoe. The canoe is sinking. There is much turnover on the unit and the unit becomes short-staffed due to its reputation. These are arguably the worst traits observed in managers. It is a big nursing world. Nurses talk and word gets around.

Truth Number Two

Most managers are phenomenal advocates for nursing staff. They choose to lead by being excellent role models of respect, kindness, compassion, and empathy for their staff members. They are present and use their intuition to sense the needs of their department and staff. They promote building their team members up to achieve their desired goals for the departments they lead. They don't tear their teams down. These managers are a safe haven and have the ability to care for their caregivers. They also exhibit the courage to call out bad behavior and consistently maintain fair consequences. They also provide opportunities for all involved to learn and grow. These managers seek to promote the individual gifts of their nurses because they know the value of the sum of the whole. They value their nurses and let them know it.

Let's say your experiences fall in the first category of nurse managers. Granted, being a manager of a unit and/or department is hard work, and managers are human and imperfect. More than likely, your manager is doing the best he or she can do under circumstances you may be unaware of and definitely not privy to. They have issues just as much as the next person, and some handle their issues better than others. You're not going to resolve *their* issues by being passive/aggressive or gossiping about them behind their backs. That behavior will only bring you misery in more ways than you could imagine. Unless you have plans to apply for their position as a manager, you need to figure out your role in contributing to a positive team experience during your shift.

If you can't align with the situation, despite controlling your own thoughts and actions, it is time to look for a position elsewhere. Staying in a situation that is toxic will only lead to your own increasing unhappiness, frustration and stress. Go back to the Golden Rule - *To thine own self be true*. Your power is in how you choose to respond to what your intuition is telling you.

I believe nurse managers wanted to start out right, but get sucked into administration not allowing them to make decisions based on their unit's needs. They lose touch with their staff and take a lot of heat from their superiors in administration. They are stuck between satisfying their staff and administrators' needs and trying to conform to make everything fit. Basically, the nurse managers have no power. There are no good options and are stuck with what they are given by admin, which leads to conformity or to leaving management all together.

— Anonymous, FL

Whether your relationship with your nurse manager falls in truth category one or two, make the effort to help your manager shine like a brilliant star. Have compassion for the demands the job entails and show gratitude for even the smallest attempt on your manager's part to make you feel special and appreciated.

Giving your manager the benefit of the doubt goes a long way toward empowering good management practices. It's your choice to make the day go smoothly or go down that slippery slope of no return by constantly undermining, sabotaging, and talking smack about your manager. That type of thinking will only deepen the poor morale and resentment towards your manager, for yourself and other teammates. Working *with* your manager expends much less of your precious energy than constantly resisting her efforts to manage a team of nurses with varied experience and skills — and personalities.

Nurse Managers are in a difficult position. They are doing more with less the days and it can really take its toll on the leaders and their spirit. I actually know several people that went into management, and like me, were ready to take on the world and make everything better. Then, when the reality of red tape and workload set in, they too left management and went back to direct patient care.

— Jeni Fitzpatrick, Oregon

This is not giving your manager a free pass for treating you or anyone else unfairly or with disrespect, or publicly shaming others into submission to follow their rules and unreasonable expectations. The writing is on the wall with that kind of behavior, and you know what you need to do: Take your gifts, passion, and commitment elsewhere to a manager who embraces and supports who you are.

An assistant nurse manager recently retired after 38 years of providing exceptional nursing care and commented on her administrative role:

I missed the actual patient care when I went into management.

— Anonymous (state omitted per request)

Jeni is a nurse who began her nursing career at the bedside, gradually working into the roles of charge nurse, then assistant nurse manager, then nurse manager, before choosing to go back to bedside nursing. She says:

I have had the rare opportunity to see and feel the important role of nurse managers in the inpatient setting. When I ultimately decided to leave management and go back to direct patient care, it was probably the biggest and most brave decision I've ever made.

I walked away from a role I was good at, a role I know I could have gone far in for a few reasons, the first being that I desperately missed the joy I felt when caring for patients. The feeling you get when you make a patient's situation or life just a little bit better. God, I missed that. I love *taking care of patients.*

A Special Note to Managers

Respect is a two-way street. Commanding respect is different from demanding respect. Treat your staff with respect, honesty, transparency (in areas you are able to), and gratitude and you will have a staff that adores and respects you. Staff will not hesitate to do anything you ask of them.

Please don't take your personal problems to work. Your staff has enough problems of their own, as well as a pretty demanding and stressful twelve hours to get through. They look to you as a beacon of light and wisdom. You are their rock.

See to it your staff gets their lunch break and other breaks. Make an effort to give them permission for self-care throughout the day.

Be observant of your staff's demeanor and intervene with kindness and compassion if they are having a rough day. Listen to their concerns and work together to find solutions that will meet the needs of your staff, unit, and administration. Caring for your caregivers will go a long way in retaining and recruiting nurses who are referred to your unit from your staff. As I said earlier, nurses talk to other nurses.

Recalling your experiences as a staff nurse will allow you to have empathy for your staff and the ability to resolve issues before they get out of control, thus affecting the entire unit.

Finally, please honor and be an advocate for your staff with hospital administration. Be fearless in providing clear understanding of what your staff experiences in the trenches, which stems from administrators' decisions that are influenced by financial outcomes.

If your actions inspire others to dream more, learn more, do more, and become more, you are a leader.

— John Quincy Adams

A patient shared:

I had an experience where the nurse was caring for my physical monitoring needs, but was not able to see how much I just needed to cry. I just needed someone to listen to me. Maybe hug me. I was scared with what was happening and I was afraid to ask for a different nurse. I became so upset with her care I asked to speak with the nurse manager. She listened without judgment and provided a nurse she thought would be a better fit. My new nurse was an angel and amazing! She actually sat down and had a conversation with me and asked what I needed and expected. I cried. She hugged me. Truly hugged me. I will be forever grateful to the compassion of that nurse manager and the nurse. My entire experience from that point on was phenomenal.

One nurse easily expressed feeling unappreciated and misunderstood more times than not on her unit:

I'm just a warm body and it seems as if I can do nothing right. Just last week, my nurse manager called me into her office (again) and wrote me up for something others had complained about concerning me. She didn't even give me a chance to share my thoughts about what they, whoever they are, went to her for. I don't feel supported by anyone, especially my manager. Why would she believe others over me? I don't fit in. I am stressed out thinking about what else she will write me up for. I hate second-guessing my patient care for twelve hours. I didn't think nursing would be like this. I'm thinking that I'm done. [The nurse disclosing her thoughts about management was adamant about anonymity.] *I'm afraid I'll lose my job. I need this job to support my daughter."* —

Anonymous, NC

This is a sad, but true commentary relative to the nurse's experience with management, which made her fear retribution. At the time of this writing, she made the painful decision to resign from her position after finding another position at a competing hospital. Fortunately, she didn't leave nursing altogether.

> *We will be known forever by the tracks we leave.*
>
> *—Dakota*

Thoughts on Management

1. How do you feel about your manager(s) and why?

2. If you are or ever have been a manager, in what ways did you support your staff?

3. What are the methods to promote honest communication which foster respect between managers and staff?

Part III

Nursing Leadership

Where *are* you? Yes, I'm calling out *you* and everyone else, regardless your management level.

Warning: *You may* not *like the mirror reflecting the reality of the current nursing climate that you have had an integral part in creating. You may even become angry and filled with adamant denial as you read.*

As nursing leaders, you have committed to the responsibility of defining the nursing profession. Holding a leadership position at the highest level of nursing commits you to honoring nurses' voices and expectations, and to accept changes that benefit nurses and their profession, as well as standing strong in safe patient care. You are the voice and action for the nurses you represent.

I have experienced change after change after change within our profession throughout my 29 years of nursing. It has come to a point where I am angry. My anger lies in the deterioration of a beautiful art form — nursing.

When did our patients become clients? How did our hospitals become money-driven corporations marketing healthcare as a business? *Seriously?*

This business mindset was nurtured and allowed to grow to a point of seemingly no return throughout the past few decades, It has deeply scarred the nursing profession in more ways than one could imagine. For example, insurance companies jumped on the bandwagon and now claim a critical place in dictating how healthcare is practiced, altering time-honored processes for making decisions about patient care and the best way to provide it.

I would like to know what happened to the "Art of Nursing."

If I remember correctly, practicing the science of nursing as an art form was the foundation of nursing. Nurses took pride as they practiced nursing from their hearts, being ever vigilant about knowing their patients' needs before summoned by a call light. Beds were made every day. Patients were bathed every day.

A nurse could actually sit down and have a nice conversation with the patients about ways to meet their needs. You know. The basic stuff. There was time for this interaction and it was considered an important part of nursing. It's called, "presence," being an authentic presence for our patients.

Presence as a nursing behavior was expected and protected. Nursing also was considered a career, not simply a job to pay the bills. Somehow, the standard of nursing has become more of a task of maintaining charting mandates, offset by shrinking actual patient care. Once again, this puts nurses in a position of proving that mandated care was done. Combined with an unrealistic—and I'm going to firmly state—unsafe nurse to patient ratio, it is no wonder the Art of Nursing has been nearly lost.

There is such a push to have minimum staffing to save money. When we had extra help, we were able to go through the unit bathing our patients, changing linens, helping with admissions, transfers and discharges. It was a happier time for all, especially the patients.

—Anonymous, FL

A solution to the current nurse to patient ratio dilemma is to hire more nurses. It is critical that nurses maintain a current knowledge of expected and recommended evidence-based guidelines from established, respected organizations that represent our interests as professional nurses. Without such standards, the issue of attracting and, more importantly, retaining those called to nursing becomes a greater problem thus further contributing to the nursing shortage.

Many studies (cited at the end of this book), have clearly demonstrated the negative impact relative to patient care as a consequence of inadequate staffing, which in turn, results in the very outcome administrators are attempting to avoid—readmission, increased liability and an inability to retain nurses. We have become mired in an endless, self-sustaining and dangerous loop.

To speak the language CEOs and administrators only seem to hear, reluctance to adequately staff units affects the financial bottom line. Most importantly, your decision to inadequately staff nurses does not meet patients' needs. And, patients will go elsewhere. Patients today are savvy, well-read, and hypervigilant about healthcare they choose to meet their needs.

No need to shoot the messenger. I am only pointing out evidence-based facts. Yes, right about now I feel the icy stare from administrators and nursing leaders as they think about the corporate bottom line.

Furthermore, and previously alluded to, we see an apparent disconnect between what nurses are taught in nursing schools versus what is actually happening when they begin their first job. Nurses who were educated and prepared to care for their patients have every reason to be disillusioned and disheartened by the lack of consistency between their education and actual practice. For nurses coming into the profession, it's the ultimate "bait and switch." It's easy to see why the current business-oriented healthcare model's effect on nursing gives those new to the profession every reason to *run*.

Nurses with integrity won't align with a system that does not put its money where its mouth is. Talk is cheap and the truth always comes out no matter the situation. It is no wonder there is a nursing shortage that is only becoming worse.

A recent new grad confided:

I am overwhelmed. Nursing school did not prepare me for the reality of what nursing is. We did a lot of case studies and role playing. What I really wish is that we would have been taught basic nursing stuff like doing IVs. I don't think the instructors know what is really happening in nursing. I am not sure nursing is for me, not since seeing how it really is. It's all about the technology. I became a nurse to care for people — vulnerable people.

— Anonymous, WV

And yet another insight:

I am so disappointed where nursing has come. I was not trained to care for patients as it is done today and I've seen many changes throughout my 40 years of practice that have undermined the very essence of nursing practice and what I know it to truly be. It breaks my heart that I cannot care for patients as I would like and they deserve. It is all about the money now. Not patient care.

— Anonymous, Oregon

Nursing administrators and managers, are you hearing your fellow nurses?

It takes a lot more than a few brief

impromptu visits to the units to make your presence known if you are unable to see the forest for the trees. You are *leaders* in nursing and you can make a difference within the nursing profession.

Please don't tell me you don't have the power because of your hospital administrators' definition of what the nurse's role is. I can only speak for myself, but I am no longer listening or believing that excuse.

It is not my intention to shame and guilt you. I only want to bring an awareness of what is going on in the trenches. I hope you will remember your "why" for becoming a nurse and take action to become a change agent that will bring the heart and voice back into nursing and healthcare.

Immediate managers are very supportive, but above that in senior leadership, those at the highest, it's all about lobbying which is not really helpful to the bedside nurses.

— Anonymous, FL

Nursing leaders are in an optimal position to design, support and create an environment within healthcare where nurses practice the art of nursing. *You* have the power to bring nursing back to what it was meant to be. Have the gumption and wherewithal to stand up and say to your administrators, "There's a better way."

You are the voice for the nursing staff. Your pivotal role defines nursing and determines how nursing is practiced based on nursing principles, not to meet the needs of other healthcare professionals and hospital administrators. Your nurses need to know you are listening to their concerns, that you have their back, and will guide them to practice the art of nursing in all healthcare areas.

Any nurse who has practiced for any length of time can relate to this candid observation:

Nursing is becoming more and more responsible for everyone. If one area doesn't do their job, it falls back on nursing.

— Anonymous, FL

Being in a leadership position means you must be *the leader*. Now is the time to use your skills, influence, and compassion for your nurses and to renew the passion for nursing.

The report, "2010 Institute of Medicine: Future of Nursing," recommended nurses take more seats on hospital boards, thereby adding a valuable voice in shaping policies affecting the future of healthcare. Unfortunately, that did not happen.

Based on the results to a survey of 1000 hospitals cited in the 2015 analysis, the percentage of nurses on hospital boards fell from 6% to %5 from 2011 to 2014, whereas physicians' percentage of seats on boards held steady at 20%.

Nurse Leaders: Be the trendsetters for the profession of nursing.

It takes immense courage as a nurse leader to be a trendsetter for the profession of nursing. It is undoubtedly a nursing role that has the potential to take nurse leaders out of their comfort zone more times than not. Great leaders are renowned for their innate ability to consistently meet the demands of the situation no matter the circumstances or discomfort. In the current healthcare climate, nurse leaders have the opportunity to truly make a difference in positively impacting nurses' roles, work environment and fair compensation.

Nurses are not playing the victim card. It is a matter of nurses needing a voice and firm representation from our nursing leaders, and you have the power to do so.

Our nursing leaders are the key to changing the current tide. My bets are on you.

We need inspired leaders. We need that excitement and that desire to propel healthcare forward.

—Jeni, Oregon

> **A good chief gives, he does not take.**
>
> **—Mohawk**

Thoughts on Inspired Leadership

1. How do you feel about nursing leadership and its impact on your current practice?

2. As a leader, what stops you from empowering your nurses' worth to hospital administrators?

3. What are the leadership qualities that will make a difference for nurses and their profession?

Afterthoughts

Feeling compassion for ourselves in no way releases us from responsibility for our actions. Rather, it releases us from the self-hatred that prevents us from responding to our life with clarity and balance.

—Tara Brach

Nurses willingly and generously give their gifts of love, passion, and service to the vulnerable every hour of every day. The time has come to generously give to themselves, thus creating a healthy work environment for themselves, staff and patients. What is your "why" and how will you carry out your passion for nursing in life? As a nurse, you have the power to change the perception of nursing by redefining the true role of the nurse.

This little book was created with the intention to give nurses validation for what they are and do as individuals and professionals. Truth be told, this book was written to light a fire in the belly of nursing professionals to redefine nursing and take back the powerful "why" that led them to seek nursing as a career. Change is indeed hard. The nursing profession has morphed, repeatedly I might add, to meet the needs of constantly changing healthcare organizations. They've adapted to change while maintaining quality and providing safe patient care, often defined by other disciplines including hospital administrators.

The following statistics may be an indicator of what the future of nursing could be if the profession continues to be defined by other financially-driven disciplines:

According to Strategic Programs, LLC 2013 research:

"…55% of RNs were over the age of 50. In 2014, the RN turnover rate was 17.2 percent, with a job

vacancy rate of 6.7 percent.

Nurses frequently change jobs — 13 percent of newly licensed RNs changed jobs after one year, and 37 percent reported that they felt ready to change jobs in the first year.

Nurse graduates report feeling pressure not to ask questions, and describe situations in which nurses with more experience often aren't willing to mentor or offer help.

Training and orientation are the second biggest issues cited by nurses as to why they left a position within the first three months. These factors, along with undesirable shift hours, high levels of job-related stress and insufficient staffing, all lead to lower job satisfaction causing many new nurses to change jobs."

Currently, nurses have the rare and wonderful opportunity to come together for a common cause, healing the healer. As nurses create new expectations based in compassionate self-care, the profession as a whole will become intolerant of overwhelm, compassion fatigue, burn-out, and illness imposed by the current unrealistic demands of the healthcare system, thus nursing can be defined as a profession that values its worth and role as medical professionals.

Making a commitment to excellence in thought, words, and action brings authenticity and integrity to self and nursing as a profession. I believe we all made that commitment as we heard and acknowledged our calling to become nurses. Some of the burning questions I've had in recent years though my experiences as a nursing professional are as follows:

Do we, as a profession, have the commitment and courage to change the perception of the current awareness and understanding of what nursing is? That question demands fortitude to defy the vision of nursing based on the perceptions and needs of other disciplines, including hospital administrators who, in my opinion, have undermined nursing and nurses for decades.

When will we gather together for a common cause to call it as we see it and take back our professional practice from a base of compassion for self?

And, finally, when will we, as nurses, define our role as we know it to be and be supported for doing so?

I'm aware that my inquiries in this book may have opened the proverbial Pandora's Box. However, this is my truth and I am standing firm in expressing it. Doubtless, some nurses don't hold the same belief, and that's fine, as I honor and respect others standing where they are within their professional journey. Our opinions are based on experiences and expectations, which may differ widely.

With that said, I'd bet many more nurses have experienced what I have described within this book and feel as I do that a change needs to occur within the profession. An underlying fear of retribution from powerful healthcare organizations is evident from the pervasive requests for anonymity from the nurses I quote in this book. When nurses sense that speaking their truth could jeopardize their careers and current positions, we're seeing another symptom of a healthcare system in crisis.

There is no time like the present to implement change—positive change—for a profession dedicated to caring for others. Now, it is time for us to graciously receive the same gifts we've generously given to others.

I wish for you the many blessings and fulfillment you undoubtedly will experience during your career as a nurse. Florence Nightingale used the light from her lamp burning to care for her patients. The light from her lamp shines upon all nurses with compassion and eternally burns with passion for our profession.

My beloved fellow nurses: I see your beauty. I see your brilliance. As long as you continue your career in nursing, shine your light to all you care for, especially to yourself. You are making a difference in our world in more ways than you imagine and are appreciated more than words could ever express. Take back your profession as it was meant to be. Remember your "why" for becoming a nurse and always, always, always compassionately care for yourself each and every day. You are worth it.

> *When we do the best we can,*
> *we never know what miracle is*
> *wrought in our life, or in the*
> *life of another.*
>
> *— Helen Keller*

Nursing Affirmations

May you always show up and be authentic, standing firm in your truth and commitment of how you define nursing.

May you be strong and fearless in letting others know your worth.

May you know your resources and how to find answers to questions about appropriate and accurate information on nursing practice.

May you have no fear to use your voice responsibly for yourself, your peers and especially your patients.

May you be the type of nurse you want to work with.

May you ask for help when you need it, no matter how old or how long you have been practicing nursing.

May you honor your patients and spend more time with them to give them the care, respect, and dignity they deserve.

May you always honor and take care of your needs. You cannot serve from an empty vessel.

May you have the wisdom and inner knowing to choose a working environment that fosters a mutually respectful relationship with management that aligns with your vision of nursing.

May you embrace the practice of compassionate self-care that is the foundation for your ability to compassionately care for others.

May you always prioritize personal and professional honesty, integrity of the highest order, and courage to stand for yourselves and others with compassion.

Acknowledgements

To Chuck Ricks, a phenomenal nurse, writer extraordinaire and dear friend. My heartfelt gratitude for the countless times you have nurtured my dreams and creativity, for being a rock during times of self-doubt, the voice of reason and wisdom, and especially for your unconditional love, support, spontaneous humor and presence in my life. You have helped my gypsy soul to soar in joy.

To the numerous nurses and nursing instructors I have had the honor and privilege to learn from and work with throughout my career. You have played an important role in making me a better nurse. I would not be the nurse I am today if our paths had never crossed. You are amazing, honored and forever cherished.

To my beautiful parents, Hazel and the late Gene Bradley, who strongly encouraged and supported me to become a nurse as a single parent. I am forever grateful for your love and flexible presence caring for your grandsons while supporting my studies. I hold deep gratitude in my heart for all you have done to support my nursing and midwifery journeys.

To Matthew and Michael, two remarkable, fine young men who are my beloved sons. You are the light in my life and have blessed me with more joy than I could have ever imagined and the clarity to know the importance of living life in the now.

To three heart-centered, amazing and brilliant women, whose shared experiences, expertise, belief in this book's message to caregivers, invaluable guidance and painstakingly hard work allowed *A Nurse's Medicine Basket* to emerge into the light as it was meant to be. My sincere gratitude to Cynthia Bryn "Cammie" Williams, fellow artist and author, Maria Connor, author and a writer's concierge and editor, author and public Speaker, Virginia McCullough for taking me under your 'Angel Wings' as a novice writer determined to bring awareness to the current challenges within the nursing profession. I am most honored to have had the opportunity to create with such beautiful spirits. Thank you for being part of making a difference in the nursing world.

A Nurse's Medicine Basket was born into being through Mother Mary, the ultimate caregiver. She is credited for the inspiration to writing this book from the heart. I am eternally grateful for her guidance in bringing an awareness of the need for compassionate self-care for all...especially our Nurses.

Tina Bradley Gain
July 2018

Statistics, Facts, and References

According to the Bureau of Labor Statistics' Employment Projections 2014-2024, Registered Nursing (RN) is listed among the top occupations in terms of job growth through 2024. The RN workforce is expected to grow from 2.7 million in 2014 to 3.2 million in 2024, an increase of 439,300 or 16%. The Bureau also projects the need for 649,100 replacement nurses in the workforce bringing the total number of job openings for nurses due to growth and replacements to 1.09 million by 2024. (http://www.bls.gov/news.release/pdf/ecopro .pdf)

Nursing Education

Master's and doctoral programs in nursing are not producing a large enough pool of potential nurse educators to meet the demand. Efforts to expand the nurse educator population are frustrated by the fact that thousands of qualified applicants to graduate nursing programs are turned away each year.

In 2016, AACN found that 9,757 qualified applicants were turned away from master's programs, and 2,102 qualified applicants were turned away from doctoral programs. The primary reasons for not accepting all qualified students were a shortage of faculty and clinical education sites. American Association of Colleges of Nursing (AACN): http://www.aacnnursing.org/News-Information/Fact-Sheets/Nursing-Faculty-Shortage

http://www.aacnnursing.org/News-Information/Press-Releases/View/ArticleId/20452/oppose-fy18-budget

Nursing Shortage Dilemma

American Association of Colleges of Nursing (AACN http://www.aacnnursing.org/news-information/nursing-shortage) reports:

According to the "United States Registered Nurse Workforce Report Card and Shortage

Forecast" published in the January 2012 issue of the *American Journal of Medical Quality*, a shortage of registered nurses is projected to spread across the country between 2009 and 2030. In this state-by-state analysis, the authors forecast the RN shortage to be most intense in the South and West. (http://ajm.sagepub.com)

Insufficient staffing is raising the stress level of nurses, which impacts job satisfaction and drives many nurses away from the profession. (www.HealthStream.com/solution-clinical development/onboard-retain-nurses)

In the December 2016 issue of *BMJ Quality & Safety*, the international journal of healthcare improvement, Dr. Linda Aiken and her colleagues released findings from a study of acute care hospitals in Belgium, England, Finland, Ireland, Spain, and Switzerland, which found that a greater proportion of professional nurses at the bedside is associated with better outcomes for patients and nurses. Reducing nursing skill mix by adding assistive personnel without professional nurse qualifications may contribute to preventable deaths, erode care quality, and contribute to nurse shortages.

In the March 2005 issue of *Nursing Economic$*, Dr. Peter Buerhaus and colleagues found that more than 75% of RNs believe the nursing shortage presents a major problem for the quality of their work life, the quality of patient care, and the amount of time nurses can spend with patients. Looking forward, almost all surveyed nurses see the shortage in the future as a catalyst for increasing stress on nurses (98%), lowering patient care quality (93%) and causing nurses to leave the profession (93%). High nurse retirement and turnover rates are affecting access to health care.

In the September 21, 2015 issue of *Science Daily*, healthcare economist David Auerbach released findings from a new study, which found that almost 40% of registered nurses are over the age of 50. "The number of nurses leaving the workforce each year has been growing steadily from around 40,000 in 2010 to nearly 80,000 by 2020. Meanwhile, the dramatic growth in nursing school enrollment over the last 15 years has begun to level off."

In September 2007, Dr. Christine T. Kovner and colleagues found that 13% of newly licensed RNs had changed principal jobs after one year, and 37% reported that they felt ready to change jobs. These findings were reported in the *American Journal of Nursing* in an article titled

"Newly Licensed RNs' Characteristics, Work Attitudes, and Intentions to Work."

Nurse Staffing

Many scientific studies point to the connection between adequate levels of registered nurse staffing and safe patient care.

In a study published in the May 2013 journal, *BMJ Quality & Safety,* researcher Heather L. Tubbs-Cooley and colleagues observed that higher patient loads were associated with higher hospital readmission rates. The study found that when more than four patients were assigned to an RN in pediatric hospitals, the likelihood of hospital readmissions increased significantly.

In the August 2012 issue of the *American Journal of Infection Control,* Dr. Jeannie Cimiotti and colleagues identified a significant association between high patient-to-nurse ratios and nurse burnout with increased urinary tract and surgical site infections. In this study of Pennsylvania hospitals, the researchers found that "increasing a nurse's patient load by just one patient was associated with higher rates of infection." The authors conclude that, "reducing nurse burnout can improve both the well-being of nurses and the quality of patient care."

In a study publishing in the April 2011 issue of *Medical Care*, Dr. Mary Blegen and her colleagues from the University of California, San Francisco found that, "higher nurse staffing levels were associated with fewer deaths, lower failure-to-rescue incidents, lower rates of infection, and shorter hospital stays."

In March 2011, Dr. Jack Needleman and colleagues published findings in the *New England Journal of Medicine*, which indicate that "insufficient nurse staffing was related to higher patient mortality rates." These researchers analyzed the records of nearly 198,000 admitted patients and 177,000 eight-hour nursing shifts across 43 patient-care units at large academic health centers. The data show that the mortality risk for patients was about 6% higher on units that were understaffed as compared with fully staffed units.

In the study titled "Nurse Staffing and Inpatient Hospital Mortality," the researchers also found that when a nurse's workload increases because of high patient turnover, mortality risk also increases.

In a study published in the April 2010 issue of *Health Services Research*, Dr. Linda Aiken and colleagues found that lower patient-nurse ratios on medical and surgical units were associated with significantly lower patient mortality rates. The study is titled "Implications of the California Nurse Staffing Mandate on Other States."

In March 2007, a comprehensive report initiated by the Agency for Healthcare Research and Quality was released on Nursing Staffing and Quality of Patient Care. Through this meta-analysis, the authors found that the shortage of registered nurses, in combination with an increased workload, poses a potential threat to quality. Increases in registered nurse staffing was associated with reductions in hospital-related mortality and failure to rescue as well as reduced length of stays. In settings with inadequate staffing, patient safety was compromised.

Levels of Education and Outcomes

In the June 2009 issue of the *International Journal of Nursing Studies*, a research team lead by Dr. Koen Van den Heede found a significant association between the number of baccalaureate-prepared RNs on cardiac care units and in-hospital mortality. Data analyzed by this international team of researcher that included representatives from Belgium, Canada, the Netherlands, and the United States showed that there were 4.9 fewer deaths per 1,000 patients on intensive care units staffed with a higher percentage of nurses with bachelor's degrees.

A growing body of research clearly links baccalaureate-prepared nurses to lower mortality and failure-to-rescue rates. The latest studies published in the journals *Health Services Research* in August 2008 and the *Journal of Nursing Administration* in May 2008, confirm the findings of several previous studies which link education level and patient outcomes. Efforts to address the nursing shortage must focus on preparing more baccalaureate-prepared nurses in order to ensure access to high quality, safe patient care.

A shortage of nurses prepared at the baccalaureate level is affecting health care quality and patient outcomes. In a study published September 24, 2003 in the *Journal of the American Medical Association (JAMA)*, Dr. Linda Aiken and her colleagues at the University of Pennsylvania identified a clear link between higher levels of nursing education and better patient outcomes. This extensive study found that surgical patients have a "substantial survival advantage" if treated in hospitals with higher proportions of nurses educated at the baccalaureate or higher degree level. In hospitals, a 10% increase in the proportion of nurses holding BSN degrees decreased the risk of patient death and failure to rescue by 5%.

Violence Against Nurses

The Joint Commission has provided results from compiling increasing incidences of violence towards nurses finding that approximately 75% of nearly 25,000 workplace assaults reported annually occurred in healthcare and social service settings.

The Joint Commission, Sentinel Event Alert: preventing violence in the healthcare setting. Issue 45, June 3, 2010; addendum, page 3, February 2017. (https://http://www.jointcommisssion.org/ass ets/1/18/SEA_45add.pdf https://www.jointcommission.org/assets/1/18 /SEA_59_workplace_violence_4_13_18 FINAL.pdf)

According to a 2014 OSHA publication,

there were 154 injuries per 10,000 workers. Within public hospital settings, 228 employees out of 10,000 occurred in nursing homes. In 2014, an astounding total of 17,000 incidents of violence within the workplace were reported, 80% of these from patients. OSHA.gov/publications/OSHA (A 3826.pdf).

Many published articles bring awareness of the increasing incidence of violence in the workplace including two outstanding references below:

https://www.nurse.com/blog/2017/08/25/workplace-violence-nurses-should-not-be-afraid-to-go-to-work/

https://health.usnews.com/health-care/for-better/articles/2017-09-29/violence-in-the-health-care-workplace.

Endorsements

A must read for nurses, nursing management and educators. The author pulls from her vast and varied professional experience and presents many imperative challenges for the future of the nursing profession.

Tina Bradley Gain delivers a clear message that nurses must take responsibility to advocate for themselves as well as their patients. Nurses need to support and nurture each other and learn to speak their truth. Healthcare delivery systems are changing to a corporate structure and nursing needs to be able to present a cohesive force to assure a strong nursing profession to face the changes and challenges in the future.

Ms. Bradley-Gain is a nurse who knows her why and speaks her truth. I have had the joy of working with her and know that she speaks from the heart in a way that resonates with her love and concerns for the profession.

—Karyn Buchanan, RNC-OB, BS-Psychology

This book is a must read. Tina Bradley Gain is both eloquent and blunt as she brings to light issues plaguing the nursing profession. I laughed, I cried and I was inspired. Tina not only calls out the things many nurses have been thinking, but are too afraid to say, but she also offers actions that can be taken to improve the profession from a multifaceted approach. This book is inspiring on many levels and I would recommend it to healthcare workers and healthcare consumers alike.

—Jeni Fitzpatrick, RNC-OB, MSN

Can a profession based upon an ethic of beneficence survive in a healthcare environment with a growing ethic based on corporate greed and avarice, and where a supererogatory expectation of personal sacrifice is demanded over the need for self-care and personal survival?

A Nurse's Medicine Basket *captures all that is both right and wrong with nursing today and provides guidance to navigate the treacherous waters of the ever expanding medical-industrial complex while staying true to the nursing ethic of caring for self, patient, colleagues and the profession.*

A Nurse's Medicine Basket *encourages nurses, young and old, to reclaim ownership of the nursing profession from this relentless onslaught before it claims nursing as its own rather than where that ownership rightly belongs, with nurses themselves.*

Speaking truth to power, Ms. Bradley-Gain offers simple yet challenging advice to salvage an overburdened profession.

Admonishing and coherent, and with the same compassion, integrity and duty to care that epitomizes the nursing profession, A Nurse's Medicine Basket *tackles some of the greatest challenges in nursing today and provides a necessary guide for all who choose the passion of nursing.*

— Robert B. Shabanowitz, PhD, HCLD (ABB)
Director, ART/Andrology Laboratory
Geisinger Medical Center, Chair Emeritus
Bioethics Review & Advisory Committee

About the Author

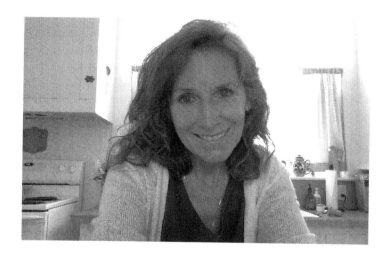

Born and raised in the Northern Tier of Pennsylvania, Tina now resides in Sayre, PA. Tina was among the students of the last diploma nursing program of the Robert Packer Hospital School of Nursing in 1989.

Her desire to become a Certified Nurse Midwife led to her first OB/GYN staff nurse position at Geisinger Medical Center in Danville, Pennsylvania. During her 14 years of employment there, Tina obtained her BSN and then MSN as she achieved her dream of becoming a Certified Nurse Midwife.

Tina began her hospital-based midwifery career in the Appalachian Mountains of West Virginia as a National Health Service Corp Scholar in 2003. In 2005, Tina landed in her beloved Oregon practicing as a CNM in several facilities including Oregon Health Science University, Kaiser Permanente NW, and Samaritan OB/GYN until 2012. Tina's midwifery Chapter in her career ended at Geisinger Medical Center as she chose to return to bedside nursing.

Currently, Tina works as a staff nurse in women's healthcare as she writes, blogs and paints preferably in nature during her days off. Her passion for the creative arts has paralleled her passion for nursing as she finds creating as another healing modality.

Her inspiration is drawn from her professional surroundings and many of Tina's writings are a result of her own nursing experiences as well as listening to the shared experiences of her fellow nurses. Throughout her almost three decades of nursing, Tina has been aware of the many changes in healthcare impacting nurses and patients. Her desire to empower every nurse's ability for self-care has provided awareness to the ongoing need for nurse advocacy in a healthcare system focused on profit.

Tina's desire to bring awareness to the current issues impacting nursing through her writing has led to a passion as a nursing advocate and giving voice to valuing nurses for the various roles they provide in healthcare. She also strongly believes in promoting nursing self-care as a priority within the work environment.

It was through working closely with other nurses that Tina observed their strength, courage, compassion, vulnerability, and commitment to patient care—often to the detriment of their own needs. These nurses have inspired her to bring awareness to the current trends in today's healthcare arena that negatively affect nurses, with the intention of creating a working environment where nurses are honored, valued, and cared for as they give care.

She believes nurses to have a crucial role as the gatekeepers of society, influencing change within the nursing profession, which positively affects our communities and the world. With this belief, Tina initiated her first blog, Nurses Heal

Thyself, to bring awareness to the realities of nursing in today's healthcare system. She offered her website as a safe container for nurses to share concerns and experiences and encourages dialogs to support nurses in becoming change agents who redefine the role of nursing, thus benefitting the nursing profession.

Bringing attention to nurses is not exclusive to Tina's writing. In 2015, Tina implemented the Community Canvas Project as an outlet for nurses to decrease stress and allow for non-verbal expression relative to their experiences as a caregiver facilitating "healing the healer."

Tina's future plans include continuing community canvas projects and offering writing/painting workshops focusing on specific topics that will facilitate individual and community healing and growth as well as continuing to write about nursing.

47739268R00096

Made in the USA
Columbia, SC
03 January 2019